MEMORIES FROM THE DEMENTIA WARD

Edward Spellman

Memories from the Dementia Ward
By Edward Spellman

Copyright © Edward Spellman 2024. All rights reserved. This book or any portion thereof may not be reproduced or used in any manner whatsoever without the express written permission of the publisher and author except for the use of brief quotations in a book review.
Edited by Lauren Elise Daniels.
Published by Edward Spellman.
A CIP catalogue record for this title is available from the Australian National Library.

ISBN- 978-1-7636927-5-6

Dedication

This book is dedicated to all the
members of staff, residents' relatives, and
anyone else who finds the reality of the
Dementia Ward challenging.

Contents

Broken Wings 1

Why I Wrote This Book 5

The Wastepaper Basket Incident 9

Shit Everywhere 15

Stray Pads 27

Using the Alcove as a Toilet 33

Gwen and the Shower Curtain 37

Ten Minutes of Comedy 39

Shoulder Charge in the Hallway 43

Throwing out $400 Worth of New Clothes 47

Gwen Flashing her Boobs 57

Farmer Pete 61

Kicking, Scratching, Punching, Spitting 67

The $5 Note..71

The Dinner Table 75

It Might Kill Me But..........................79

Shoes, Hat, and Pat 85

Fighting with Brian............................87

Hiding Behind the Foyer Curtains 97

There, Take That 101

Punched in the Face 107

Strawberry Jam 111

Folding in the Dark 115

Scooching Along the Corridor Floor 121

Cornering a Visitor in the Foyer 131

Fake Fainting in the Hallway..........135

Hiding in the Wardrobe....................141

No Sleep..145

Fifty Cents......................................151

A Trail of Poo..................................155

Gwen Peeing in my Glove 167

Don't you mean Paul.......................169

Broken Wings

I worked in aged care for twenty years, the last six and a half in a locked dementia ward. In the dementia ward I worked the afternoon shift, 2:30 to 10:30 five days a week. One day as I passed my supervisors office, she called me in and asked, "How do you handle working in the dementia ward?"

"I see the people in the dementia ward as angels with broken wings," I told her. "I'm just there to look after them until they're ready to go home."

The dementia ward was a pretty stressful workplace and what I said was true. During my time there, I was shat on, peed on, spewed on, and bled on. I was punched, slapped, kicked, and had a resident try to scratch my eyes out. I was attacked with knives, including a large carving knife. Forks, tables, chairs, ornaments, and food were thrown at me, including hot and cold beverages. I have also been bitten by people with their dentures in, and some without. I have been verbally attacked

Memories from the Dementia Ward

and abused by both residents and their relatives.

At the time, I was writing my memoir Uriel's Gift that was just as stressful, if not more, than working there. In some strange way that I don't really understand, the stress from working in the dementia ward cancelled out some of the stress from writing the memoir; and writing the memoir cancelled out some of the stress of working in the dementia ward, making both easier to manage.

At times when the stress was building on the job and it was raining, I would go outside and just stand with my arms outstretched and my face pointed toward the sky for a couple of minutes. That always helped.

Other times, I would hide in a resident's room with the door locked for a few minutes and just breathe. I used that one a lot. I closed my eyes and took a few deep breaths and then I was right back out into it.

After six years, I didn't last much longer working in the dementia ward once Uriel's Gift was published but these are the stories that I feel need telling.

Memories from the Dementia Ward

Why I Wrote This Book

One of the things that bothered me most was the reactions to the dementia ward by some of the new staff and residents' relatives. A bit of culture shock, I guess you could call it. It was hard to watch, and I wanted to do something about it. What I saw in these reactions were expectations not being met—expectations that could never be met.

Edward Spellman

Through my work, I found an information gap between general beliefs and the reality of the dementia ward. I wrote this book to add something from my personal experience and hopefully to alleviate some of the discomfort I've seen over the years. The dementia ward can be a scary and stressful space so with a little personal insight, I hope to help people make the transition into the world of dementia a little easier for some.

During my research phase, I asked as many people as I could what they thought of the idea of a book like this. Every single one of them said that

Memories from the Dementia Ward

they would have found their entry into the realm of dementia easier if they had had access to another perspective like this.

To that end, I've put together a selection of my experiences—that I hope will assist you in your foray into dementia—whatever that may be. To protect the privacy of the residents and their families, I have changed all the names of those mentioned in this book.

Edward Spellman

Memories from the Dementia Ward

The Wastepaper Basket Incident
Mrs Gwen Stapleton

Over the six years, I worked in the dementia ward within an aged care facility, I came to understand that it was the hardest ward to support, but eventually, I developed a routine that worked for me. I learnt how to read signs and trust my intuition, and could often stop disasters before they happened.

Edward Spellman

In my job I had to be versatile and adaptable as the situations demanded. Flexibility was the key to success.

It was pretty scary working at first, but got better at reading the residents' moods and body language. I always started out with a plan for my shift, while I also assumed that everything that could go wrong, would go wrong. Then there were the days when it was not advantageous to have a plan at all, and I just had to wing it. I suppose you could call it being in tune with the dementia ward. And that definitely helped.

Memories from the Dementia Ward

This little piece of history contained in the first chapter happened in my second week, when I was still very nervous about constantly tracking the residents' locations. I was organising the residents for the evening meal and had come up one short. Mrs Gwen Stapleton was missing. I stood in the middle of the dining room and went over the places I had already looked but couldn't work out where she might be. Taking a deep breath, I prepared to work my way from one end of the building to the other looking for her.

As I turned to go, I saw a pair of legs from the knee down poking out from between the resident's fridge and a cupboard. There was just enough space there to fit a wastepaper basket, so that's where we kept it.

Attached to those legs was a pair of shiny black shoes that I recognised. Gwen was sitting in the wastepaper basket - very still and quiet.

I got closer for a better look.

With her hands clasped together, she was hunched down like she was hiding. She looked up at me with a cheeky grin on her face.

"Hello Gwen, would you like some soup?" I held out my hands to her.

Memories from the Dementia Ward

Gwen never spoke, she just smiled and took my hands and pulled herself up. I walked her to her table and sat her down to a nice bowl of pumpkin soup.

I knew by now that I had to start Gwen off with her meals or she would just get up and wander. I gave her one spoonful of soup, handed her the spoon, and she would finish it herself.

Then I had to make sure that the main course was ready to be put in front of her just as she finished her soup or she would be off. It was the same for dessert and for her cup of tea after. And all the while serving nineteen other

Edward Spellman

people—half a dozen of whom needed full assistance with their meals. And another couple that were just as liable to get up and go in the middle of their meal as Gwen was.

Memories from the Dementia Ward

Shit Everywhere
Miss Millicent Frobisher

One evening, I was walking back to the office after getting the last resident into bed when as I walked past Room 16, Miss Frobisher's room, and smelled that tell-tale scent. Foregoing the office or entering the room to check the source, I headed straight to the pan room where we kept the dirty laundry ready to be picked up and the bags to put it in. It also had a machine that cleans bedpans.

From there, I collected several large black plastic bags intended for anything with faeces on it, so the laundry staff would know not to put their hands on soiled linen. Next, I collected the linen trolley because I was sure I needed it so wouldn't run out of the necessary supplies before I finished cleaning up whatever was making that smell.

With supplies in hand, I got a plastic apron from the cupboard and put it on—it covered me from knee to neck. I had a funny feeling I was going to

Memories from the Dementia Ward

need it. Then I put on a paper facemask and rubber gloves, two gloves on each hand.

After delivering the black plastic bags and the linen trolley to the room, I went looking for the hoist, a small crane designed to lift people.

Ready to assess the situation, I knew my shift partner had already left about half an hour earlier, so I was on my own. Being on my own in a locked dementia ward with twenty residents was a recipe for some interesting evenings.

Turning on the lights in Miss Frobisher's room illustrated that my preparations had been necessary. There was shit everywhere.

Miss Frobisher was a tall woman with long, skinny arms and legs. Her bed was placed with the left-hand side against the wall and both sides had the bedrails up.

This evening, she had been incontinent of faeces, shoved both her hands inside her pad, had taken them out, and had gotten a little artistic: there was faeces on the wall everywhere within her reach.

I used to carry a small bottle of eucalyptus oil with me at work for just such occasions, so I put a little up both

Memories from the Dementia Ward

nostrils to cancel out some of rank odour.

As I got closer, I could see that the bedhead and bedrails were smeared with faeces. The pillowcase, bedspread, blankets, top sheet, bottom sheet, draw sheet, and plastic mac were all covered. And not just a little.

A plastic mac is a piece of heavy plastic sheet about a metre wide and long enough to tuck under both sides of the mattress. A waterproof barrier, it stops moisture from getting through to the sheet, mattress protector, and mattress. A draw sheet is about the same size but made out of heavy cotton and designed to soak up wetness as well. It's easily changed without having to remake the bed.

Miss Frobisher was covered in it. She had waste on her hands and smeared up her arms. It was in her hair, on her face, and in her ears. Her nightdress was soaked in it at the back and smeared with it at the front. We have a scale in the industry where number one is a bit like rabbit poo and number seven is watery with no solids. This was a six, watery with a little body in it. And it stank.

First off, I put her blankets and bedspread into a black plastic bag and

Memories from the Dementia Ward

tied it up. Then I moved a chair close to the bed and sat a bowl of warm soapy water on it from the bathroom.

I closed my eyes for a minute and rehearsed in my mind what I thought would be the best way to go about this without ending up as covered as Miss Frobisher was. She was quite mobile with her arms and legs floundering about. Completely lost in her dementia, she tended to grab anything or anyone that came within reach and I had to clean up her wall, and her bed, change the bed, as well as clean and change her while keeping away from her grasping hands.

Her hands were the most dangerous part of her, so I gave them a good wash before attending to her hair, face, neck, and ears. I had put a towel under her head and replaced it with a clean one when it was done. While I was doing that, her hands had been wandering so I washed them again.

I took her nightdress off and removed her continence pad and the stretch pants designed to hold it in place. Then I slipped four towels under her, two from the left and two from the right so that I had a clean workspace.

I washed and dried her hands again. Then I washed her arms, legs, and body. Then I quickly hooked her up to the hoist and transferred her into her princess chair. It's sort of a mix between a bed and a chair on wheels designed to be comfortable, stable and safe. I had covered it with a sheet and when I had her in position, I covered her with a blanket.

That left me free to strip the bed and clean the bedrails. Then the bedhead, and several other parts I found that had faeces smeared on them.

Next came the wall.

After cleaning all that up, I remade the bed and put it back in position.

I spread some more towels on the bed and did the transfer in reverse.

With Miss Frobisher on the bed, and with everything else clean, I gave her another wash because there were bits I had missed before. I replaced her continence pad and net pants then removed the extra towels from under her.

After a full hour attending to Miss Frobisher, all that remained to do was to put on her nightie, raise the bedrails, and take six large black plastic bags full of smelly stuff to the pan room. I needed to put away the linen trolley and peel off my plastic armour.

Memories from the Dementia Ward

I said goodnight to her and, exhausted, she drifted off to sleep.

Even though I had opened the bedroom windows and after finishing I sprayed her room and the hallway close to it with odour counteractant—several times—it didn't work. Even with eucalyptus oil in my nostrils, I could still smell it for the rest of the night. And for the next three days I could taste it in the back of my throat.

Edward Spellman

Memories from the Dementia Ward

Stray Pads

In the dementia ward, it's surprising how many people threw their used pads into the toilet and then flushed. Another fairly common occurrence was for residents to be embarrassed by being incontinent, so they hid their soiled pads. The most common place to hide them was the back of a drawer, usually with something in front to conceal them. If I walked into a room and smelled that tell-tale stale urine smell, it was time to go through that resident's drawers looking for used pads.

I stepped up to the door, tapped in the security code and the magnetic lock clicked open. After stepping through the door, I stopped and waited for the lock to reengage, then stepped into the hallway. The first thing I noticed was a soiled pad hanging off the handrail outside room six.

I got a pair of gloves from the closest wash station a plastic bag from the nearest resident's room. I put on the gloves, put the pad in the plastic bag, removed the gloves and put them in

Memories from the Dementia Ward

with the pad then tied up the bag. Then I was off to the pan room to dispose of the bag and wash my hands.

Into the staff room and I was still forty minutes early for my shift. I made a cup of tea while I waited. I liked getting to work early. It gave me time to get my head into the game.

That same day after the evening meal was finished and I was taking Mrs Allan to the toilet, I discovered that one of the residents had put their pull-up pad in her toilet and tried to flush it, so the toilet was blocked. Pull-ups are absorbent and rather messy after being soaked in a toilet for a while.

Edward Spellman

At that time of day, none of the maintenance crew were available and if I called the after-hours number, I would be told to call a plumber who would promise to be there first thing in the morning.

I had been down that road before.

Theoretically, I should have left it for the plumber but nothing in a dementia ward works the way it should.

Mrs Allan had dementia and still used the toilet herself although she needed help. If I had left the situation for the plumber, she would flush it for sure and cause it to overflow.

Memories from the Dementia Ward

So, I cleaned it myself. First, I put two rubber gloves on each hand. Second, I got four plastic garbage bags and doubled them by putting one inside the other to make two of those. I positioned one so I could put the yucky stuff in it and stuck my arm inside the other.

Next came the fun part where I got to scoop all of the pad that had partially broken up out of the toilet and into the waiting bag. I tied up the bag once I had scooped everything out and flushed. Then I disposed of the bag and gloves and washed my hands.

Edward Spellman

Memories from the Dementia Ward

Using the Alcove as a Toilet
Mrs Bonnie Allan

I looked after Bonnie, a wonderful little Scottish lady for a few years. She was small, feisty, wore glasses, and found interesting places to use as a toilet.

One night after everyone was in bed, I was going around checking on them. When I saw Bonnie go out the door at the end of the corridor, I headed up that way to bring her back to bed or to give her a cup of tea if she was restless.

When I opened the door to a small space surrounded by three lattice doors, there was Bonnie, squatting and peeing in the alcove.

The door into the dementia ward was not locked but the other three were. One led to the front garden and stayed locked most of the time because the footing out there was irregular and dangerous for the residents. One led to the back garden, and it was only locked at night or when the weather was particularly bad. The residents had free access to that garden during the day.

Memories from the Dementia Ward

The fourth door was locked at all times. It was the main access to the ward on that side of the building and had a keypad and magnetic lock. It was a bit like an air lock: residents could get into it from the dementia ward but could only get out by going back into the dementia ward.

Not the spot to be peeing in.

I got Bonnie up and took her back down to the dining room where I gave her a cup of tea.

Then I went and got a bucket of water and flushed the alcove.

When Bonnie was in bed, her bathroom light was on and the toilet was right there where she could see it. She had to walk past it to leave her room but still regularly ended up in the alcove to pee.

After that, if I saw Bonnie headed for the alcove, I intervened and took her to the toilet. Sometimes I caught her in time; sometimes I didn't.

Memories from the Dementia Ward

Gwen and the Shower Curtain
Mrs Gwen Stapleton

I couldn't find Mrs Stapleton……again. I searched for her from one end of the ward to the other but I couldn't locate her. The first time I went looking without turning the bedroom or bathroom lights on.

Halfway through my second run, with the lights turned on, I found the same black shoes poking out from the bottom of a shower curtain that had been poking out from behind the fridge when she was sitting in the waste paper basket. I quickly discerned that Gwen had grabbed the shower curtain and while holding it done several full turns, so she was wrapped up tight.

After I untangled her, she wore the same cheeky grin as before.

I suspected that she loved to play hide and seek when she was a child because that's how old the cheeky grin looked.

Memories from the Dementia Ward

Ten Minutes of Comedy
Mr Patrick Kelly

Mr Patrick Kelly was one hundred and ninety-eight centimetres tall, lanky, with a long narrow face and had been really angry for his first week in the dementia ward. He had difficulty communicating verbally and simply wouldn't talk, although he understood us well enough.

It was getting close to Christmas, and I found Pat in the lounge watching an old black-and-white comedy sketch on the television. The sketch only lasted about ten minutes but the change in Pat was phenomenal.

Aggressive since coming into the ward, Pat now emerged from wherever he had been hiding inside himself.

I watched him, stunned at the joy in his face and his raucous laughter as he slapped his thigh. Tears of laughter streaming down his face.

Nothing we had tried had gotten through to him. We had tried occupational therapy, music, art, games with groups. Games with just one other person. One on one chats. It all just

Memories from the Dementia Ward

made him angry. Until that sketch on the television.

When the sketch was finished Pat wiped the tears from his face, looked up at me, and mimed having a cup of tea.

After that little miracle, Pat was a different man. He interacted with other residents and staff and seemed happy most of the time and started using his own form of sign language. I didn't see him get angry again and he settled in as though he had been there for years. All due to ten minutes of comedy.

Forever after, Patrick was a true gentleman.

Edward Spellman

Memories from the Dementia Ward

Shoulder Charge in the Hallway
Mr John Ryan

I was walking up the hallway on my way to Room 6 to check in on Bonnie when Mr Ryan was walking in the opposite direction headed toward the dining room. As he approached, he brought his elbow into his body, dropped his shoulder, and lunged at me with a shoulder charge.

Edward Spellman

I knew John liked a bit of a scuffle, saw it coming, and spun out of the way.

John lost his balance and staggered into the wall as I grabbed hold from behind to help him regain his balance.

Once he had his balance he just laughed and carried on down the hallway.

A little while later in the dining room, I had to step in between John and Mrs Allan who had inadvertently gotten in front of him. The fists would come up and he would start swinging at anyone that came within arm's length.

Memories from the Dementia Ward

John was someone we needed to watch carefully, although, when he knew we were watching he behaved. The trick was to have him believe that we were watching all the time, and managed to keep him out of trouble. Well, some of it.

Edward Spellman

Memories from the Dementia Ward

Throwing out $400 Worth of New Clothes
Mrs Sophia Ruiz

Thursdays were laundry days, and one of my first tasks for the afternoon to evening shift (2:30 to 10:30) was delivering the resident's clothes to their rooms. Several of the residents were perpetually worried about whether all of their clothes had come back. One resident in particular, Mrs Sophia Ruiz got herself routinely distressed that her items had not been returned.

Sophia regularly took me to her room to show me that she did not have enough clothes and asked where the rest were. Most of her clothes were also quite old and beginning to grow threadbare. In the dementia ward, residents often got soiled and had their clothes changed several times during a shift and the regular washing took a toll on the items.

Sophia's son Theo visited regularly and she complained to him about her situation as well. Theo asked me to check her wardrobe and make a

Memories from the Dementia Ward

list of what I thought she might need, so I did.

Theo bought $400 worth of clothes for his mum, and brought them in the following day. He was worried about clothes disappearing, so he made sure he brought them when I was on shift and handed them personally to me with a request that I have them sent to the laundry to be named. With over four hundred residents throughout the facility, most of their clothing went through the onsite laundry and had to be labelled accordingly.

I bagged the new clothes in clear plastic bags and tagged the bags with,

Edward Spellman

"Please name for Mrs Ruiz" And sent them to the laundry. When the laundry attached name tags, they did it well and the tags stayed on. When residents' families attached name tags, they often did not last.

The new clothes, all with fresh name tags, came back the following Thursday and I put what needed hanging in Sophia's wardrobe, then the nighties, underpants, and singlets, into her drawers.

I went and found Mrs Ruiz and took her to show her the new clothes her son had bought for her, thinking she would be pleased.

Memories from the Dementia Ward

Never assume what's going to happen in a dementia ward.

As I started to show her the new clothes, she said, "Not my clothes."

"Yes, they are. Your son bought them for you."

"He no buy clothes for me. I buy own clothes. Take away."

This went on for about ten minutes with Mrs Ruiz taking all of the new clothes out of her wardrobe and drawers, and me putting them back and trying to convince her that they were hers.

I left her in her room and went to attend to other duties for a bit, then went to check on her about half an hour later. All of the new clothes were piled onto the end of her bed.

I tried showing her that all of these new clothes had her name on them. And again, reassuring her that her son had bought them for her but she was having none of it.

That first night, I put her clothes away about six times.

I had the next two days off and I returned to discover that a lot of the new clothes were missing.

After some investigation, I discovered that one of the other staff had found a big pile of Sophia's clothes

Memories from the Dementia Ward

outside the pan room and had sent them to the laundry. The pan room was locked and only accessible to staff.

The next Thursday, they all came back from the laundry. And again, I put them all away where they were meant to be.

I was operating from the point of view that if I just kept putting her clothes back into her wardrobe and dressing her in her new clothes, eventually she would accept them.

That didn't work. It didn't work at all.

When a staff member dressed her in her new clothes she would go back to her room and change into clothes that she recognised as her own—always the old clothes she complained about.

I didn't notice at first, but the amount of clothing in her wardrobe was decreasing. Then one day, when she thought no one was looking, I saw her with a couple of pieces of clothing under her arm walking down the corridor. I kept my eyes on her thinking she was going to put them into the laundry skip to send them off to be washed, but she bypassed the laundry and put them into the rubbish bin.

Memories from the Dementia Ward

I took them out after she had left and sent them to the laundry to be washed.

Over the next couple of weeks, that happened several times until, about three months after he had bought them, her son came to me asking about the $400 worth of clothes he had bought. He had just checked his mother's wardrobe and none were there. Every single piece had disappeared.

I had to tell him that his mother did not recognise the clothes as hers and refused to accept that he had bought them for her. Even though he had also been telling her that for three months and I had caught her several times throwing out the new clothes and redirected her. Sophia was a very strong woman determined to have her own way.

And she still complained daily about not having enough clothes.

Memories from the Dementia Ward

Gwen Flashing her Boobs
Mrs Gwen Stapleton and
Mr Patrick Kelly

Patrick was much better after getting to watch comedy sketches occasionally and was usually very polite with the ladies, so I called him Gentleman Pat.

Gwen was a small, skinny, eighty-five-year-old woman.

Edward Spellman

I was working in the dining room setting up for the evening meal while Pat watched TV just off to the side

Gwen was wandering around doing nothing in particular.

Pat sat, knees and feet spread wide in one of the single lounge chairs, looking comfortable and engrossed in his show.

I looked over toward the TV area just as Gwen walked up to Pat and stood between his knees.

Pat had lost his temper a few times in his first two weeks and each time, he had attacked someone. He hadn't since watching the comedy

Memories from the Dementia Ward

sketch but I was still wary of any of the other residents getting too close to him. He had only been there for a couple of weeks and while the television shows helped, he was still adjusting.

I was on my toes ready to react if he took offence from Gwen being too close and invading his personal space when she grabbed the bottom of her shirt and pulled it up to her neck.

No bra just boobs right in Pat's face.

His eyes went wide and his jaw dropped. I think mine did too.

Gwen just stood there with her top up as high as she could get it and

Gentleman Pat didn't seem to mind. He just sat there with a big grin on his face and watched the TV, a little happier after Gwen's little show.

Memories from the Dementia Ward

Farmer Pete

Mr Peter Brown

Mr Brown lived in the same corridor where Pat had his room. Like Pat, he often wore a hat, his Akubra, and had also been a farmer, but that's where their similarities ended.

Peter was as unlike Gentleman Pat as chalk was different from cheese. He was in a bad mood when he woke up, not particularly happy during the day, in a bad mood when he went to bed, and much the same throughout the night.

He complained about absolutely everything. I must admit though, he was pretty good at it. I thought he was possibly the best complainer I had ever met in my life.

He would complain if someone made too much noise and would make more noise than everybody he complained about. He would upset everyone in the lounge room and then go off to his room.

He would press his emergency buzzer to have his ceiling fan turned on.

Memories from the Dementia Ward

Then ten minutes later he would buzz to have it turned off.

He would buzz and complain that his bed had not been made. So, I would make his bed.

Ten or fifteen minutes later he would buzz again to complain that his bed had not been made, after pulling it apart.

After dark, he would complain that the bathroom light kept him awake. So, I would turn it off.

Then he would buzz and say that he needed the bathroom light on so he could find his way to the bathroom if he needed to.

Edward Spellman

Then there were not enough blankets, or too many. Or, I want a singlet on. Then I want it off.

He would go to bed after having been taken to the toilet and seem to settle down. Half an hour later he would turn up in the dining room without his pyjama bottoms. We would take him back to his room and find that he had peed in the corner of his bedroom.

He did this so often that no matter what we did, his bedroom stank of stale urine.

And he knew where the bathroom was but he didn't like using it.

Memories from the Dementia Ward

If he needed to use his bowels during the day, he would go out into the garden and poop under a particular tree where he could squat while leaning on the back fence.

Once we fitted his room with a laser sensor, we knew when he got out of bed and we grew more adept at getting him to the toilet.

Most of the time.

Edward Spellman

Memories from the Dementia Ward

Kicking, Scratching, Punching, Spitting

Mrs Ava Bouchard

One particular young woman in our care, Mrs Ava Bouchard, suffered from early onset Alzheimer's disease and had grown completely lost in her dementia. She believed that she didn't need any help although she couldn't walk, couldn't feed herself, couldn't toilet herself, and needed to be transferred with a hoist.

Edward Spellman

Ava got angry when anyone attempted to help her in any way. She spat food and drink into our faces while we helped her with her meals. It was safer to work from beside her ear, as she couldn't quite turn that far, but I lost concentration occasionally and drifted into range. Every time, I ended up with food on my face.

To toilet her, we had to lift her with the hoist to put her on the commode. We had to keep away from her hands because she would scratch us if she could. While up in the hoist she would lash out with either an open hand for a slap or a closed fist for the punch.

Memories from the Dementia Ward

One night, I ended up with three decent-sized scratches down my right cheek. Knowing what she may have had under her fingernails, I hit them with alcohol wipes to avoid infection.

One evening, while getting her ready for bed, she was up in the hoist when I noticed a look in her eyes.

I yelled, "Get back," to my partner but I was too late.

Ava lashed out with her foot and caught my partner right in the mouth.

It was a good, strong kick that knocked my partner back a couple of steps and split her lip.

Edward Spellman

And the truth is, nothing about this was unusual in any way. It was just what was normal for this particular resident.

Memories from the Dementia Ward

The $5 Note
Mrs Doris Cooper

Mrs Doris Cooper was often stressed about money. Before moving into the dementia ward, she had been a pensioner with no assets. Her only income was the aged pension and she always ran out of money before pension day.

I would often see her checking her purse to make sure she had some money on her. She carried a black handbag and took out her purse every few minutes to check. Someone had given her a five dollar note which kept her calm for a couple of minutes when she checked and found it.

Still, she repeated this behaviour again and again throughout all of my shifts. If she misplaced her handbag, her distress escalated very quickly and there was no way to calm her down until the purse was found and she saw the money inside.

She would take out her five dollar note, open it, and reassure herself that she had money. Then she would fold it

Memories from the Dementia Ward

several times and tuck it safely back into her purse.

That note had been folded so many times that she had worn the ink and made part of it near transparent.

After watching her fold that note for the better part of six years, I swapped it for a new one. I still have the old one and intend to mount it on a black felt background and hang it on my wall as a reminder of Doris and her worries.

Doris was also partial to a lolly or two. If she had some in her room, she was always much calmer than if she didn't so I made sure there were always lollies for her. Whenever I went on holiday, I would always make sure there was enough stock to keep her going while I was away. About a handful a day was a good measure, with the rest kept in the office so she couldn't overindulge.

Memories from the Dementia Ward

The Dinner Table
Mrs Gwen Stapleton

One evening, I was in the dining room with my partner for the dinner shift. We served from a small separate kitchen, taking food out and used dishes back in. Five residents sat at the table closest to the kitchen. Two on one side, two on the other, and one sat at the end closest to the kitchen door.

I had just cleared that table of empty soup bowls, dropped them off in the kitchen, and returned out to collect them from the next table.

Mrs Stapleton, who had been sitting quietly at her table, had taken off her shoes and socks, as well as her slacks, her net pants, and her pad and stretched out on the table of five residents.

While it wasn't surprising that she had stripped herself as she had done that several times before, it was surprising that she had managed to undress in so short a time. And still have time to climb onto the table and lie down neatly without disturbing any of the place settings. She didn't even spill

Memories from the Dementia Ward

a glass of water as she lay in the middle of five of them.

Gwen wasn't someone who could still understand requests let alone comply with them.

Rather than wasting my time asking her to get off the table I just picked her up and lifted her into her chair where I redressed her and proceeded with serving the meal.

Edward Spellman

Memories from the Dementia Ward

It Might Kill Me But
Mrs Charlotte Jackson

Charlotte was American and had a noticeable southern drawl. She was also one of my favourite residents, a gorgeous lady and a gentlewoman.

Before I helped her to sit up in bed, I counted to give her time to prepare herself.

But not one, two, three, go.

I would count, one, two, three, seven.

My excuse to her was that my way of counting was more efficient and got me there faster.

In her slow southern drawl, Charlotte told me, "You can't count. I'm going to teach you how to count," and this little game went on for a couple of months.

Then, one day when I was sitting her up on the side of her bed, I suggested that she count this time.

She said, "One, two, three, seven. Oh! Gosh darn."

It had taken me about three months to get a rapport going with

Memories from the Dementia Ward

Charlotte. And in the end, it was all due to my poor counting skills.

Each night, after Charlotte ate her dinner, she sat patiently, spoon in hand, waiting for her ice cream. It didn't matter what other types of deserts were available. Charlotte just wanted ice cream.

And I would tease her about it, telling her that all of the workers in the ice cream factory had gone on strike and there was a country-wide shortage. Or that the ice cream factory had been blown up by terrorists.

And she would say, "Where's my ice cream?"

And I would give her a bowl of ice cream.

One day I put a bowl in front of her with a teaspoon of ice cream sitting a little forlornly in the bottom of the bowl.

She looked at the tiny amount of ice cream. Then she looked up at me. Then down at the ice cream. Then up at me again. Then down at the teaspoon of dessert and said, "Well, I guess it is ice cream."

As she spooned that into her mouth, I gave her the bowl I had been hiding behind my back. It was loaded. I had filled it up as much as I could without it overflowing.

Charlotte looked at the bowl filled with ice cream. Then she looked up at me. The back at the bowl. She took a deep breath and said, "It might kill me, but I'm going to eat it all."

I wish I could write in her accent. It was gorgeous.

It took her a while, but she ate it all. She was the last person in the dining room that night and went to bed a very happy woman.

Edward Spellman

Memories from the Dementia Ward

Shoes, Hat, and Pat
Mr Patrick Kelly

One evening, I was in the office doing paperwork. It was getting late and my shift would finish in half an hour at 10:30 pm. Then I thought I heard footsteps.

The office was positioned in such a way that you could slide out the door on the office chair and get a view right down one of the main corridors. So, I rolled out the door to see whose footsteps I was hearing.

And there was Patrick, strolling down the corridor. All one hundred and ninety-eight centimetres and, what looked like another twenty centimetres of Pat swinging in the wind.

He was wearing his hat—an Akubra, of course—and his slippers. Good to see. We spent a lot of time asking people not to walk around without something on their feet to keep them from slipping.

And that was his entire ensemble for his evening stroll. Shoes, hat, and Pat.

Memories from the Dementia Ward

Fighting with Brian
Mr Brian Jones

Changing and cleaning Brian was always an interesting experience. He didn't like it one little bit.

While he was good-natured and cooperative for everything else, getting changed when he had been incontinent was challenging as he believed that he did not need to have his pad changed, or even to change his clothes when they were soiled.

Edward Spellman

When trying to take Brian to the toilet, he cooperated right up until I got him into the bathroom. Then—well, that's when things got interesting.

Luckily for us, by the time Brian moved in we had gotten more staff in the ward. We started with two, moved up to three, and then to four and sometimes it took all four of us to change him and get him cleaned up.

One day, I walked past Brian in the living room and smelled that he had been incontinent with faeces. Suspecting I would have trouble getting him changed myself, I went looking for help.

Memories from the Dementia Ward

I asked two women I was working with to wait where Brian would not be able to see them while I brought him down to his room. If we had all gone with him to his room, he would have freaked out and we had learnt that from experience.

Brian came with me to his room with no trouble and even came voluntarily into the bathroom. I then asked him if I could check his pad. He didn't know what I was talking about, so I pulled the back of his trousers out a bit and had a peek.

Just as I thought, lots of poo.

I said, "Come and sit on the toilet for me, Brian."

I tried to help him down with his trousers, but he wouldn't let me. He grabbed hold of them with both hands and locked on.

Then I asked my two colleagues to come in and help. We had tried all sorts of ways to get Brian to allow us to help him but all to no avail. The problem was that he believed that he was perfectly capable of looking after himself and that he was in no way incontinent.

He simply believed that he didn't need any help. And he was strong.

Memories from the Dementia Ward

The resident's ensuites were not very big. That small space had a shower recess, a toilet, and a hand basin. The available floor space beside those would not be much more than a square metre.

Into that space, we often squeezed four people, changed Brian, washed him, got a clean pad, and clean clothes on him. With the other two there to help, we got started.

First, we had to position him facing the hand basin. We had to be very careful while changing Brian because he kicked, bit, spat, and punched if we gave him the opportunity. Oh, and the swearing. He was rather good at that.

To get Brian's trousers down, two of us needed to take control of his hands while he would try to break our fingers. From the damage he did to her fingers, one of the staff had to take six weeks off work after helping change Brian. Keeping his hands under control meant controlling his arms and never letting him get hold of our hands.

I weigh around 75kg and Brian could slap me bodily against the wall while I was holding onto one of his arms. The other side was a little easier

Memories from the Dementia Ward

because the staff members there could wedge themselves against the wall.

The third person's job was to get his pants down, get him clean, insert a new pad, and pull it all up again. Sounds simple.

It wasn't.

Brian would spread his legs to try and keep us from getting his pants down. It often took a concerted effort from all three of us even while we struggled to maintain a hold on his arms.

Once his trousers were down and we could get him cleaned up, Brian continued to swear, and tried to kick and punch. We had to stay in a position where he couldn't spit in our faces because if he could, he would.

Once we got Brian changed and cleaned, we had to be careful as we let go because the instant we did, if he could, he delivered a punch or kick.

If we stepped out of the way fast enough, all would be good with Brian and he would tell us that it felt good and he would thank us for cleaning him up. And every time we had to clean him up it made me feel sick and disgusted with myself.

I used to pride myself on finding a way to form a rapport with the people

Memories from the Dementia Ward

I was looking after and here I was causing grief to someone who couldn't understand what was going on.

Ultimately, Brian was one of the main reasons I left the dementia ward after six and a half years. I just couldn't do it anymore.

Edward Spellman

Memories from the Dementia Ward

Hiding Behind the Foyer Curtains

Mrs Gwen Stapleton

Everyone was in bed except Mrs Stapleton and I couldn't find her anywhere. We had rules about how long we could wait before reporting a resident missing but I was positive she hadn't gotten out of the building.

Still, I checked hallways, the dining and lounge areas, and then the foyer. I searched the laundry and pan room, and the two toilets in the main area and the enclosed back garden. I couldn't find Mrs Stapleton.

Next, I checked all twenty bedrooms and bathrooms without turning the lights on to avoid disturbing anyone.

There was still no sign of Gwen, so I did it all again. Although with the lights on this time, and again I couldn't find her.

I got a torch and checked the back garden again. No Mrs Stapleton.

Four times I searched that place from one end to the other. Nothing.

Memories from the Dementia Ward

Then I was standing in the foyer wondering what to do next. The foyer is pretty big with half a dozen lounge chairs and a round table with four chairs. The lights were on and I had just checked behind all the chairs that could hide a small person.

The foyer poked out a bit from the main building and had half-height corner windows at the front with heavy full-length curtains.

I wracked my brain as my eyes wandered. Then, right in the corner, only just visible between two lounge chairs, I saw the toes of two shiny black shoes. Gwen Stapleton's shoes.

That meant that either she had hidden her shoes behind the curtain and disappeared into thin air or, she was standing quietly in the corner behind the curtains playing hide and seek again.

I pulled the curtains aside and there was Mrs Stapleton, standing still and quiet with her hands clasped together, wearing her cheeky grin.

Memories from the Dementia Ward

There, Take That
Mrs Betty Cartwright

Sometimes, I worked a morning shift, 6:30 am to 1:30 pm, when most of the showers were usually don.

One morning, I had just finished my second shower when one of the other staff came to me and said, "Can we do a swap? You do Betty and I'll do anyone you want."

I said, "Betty doesn't like me. Every time I go near her, she screams rape."

Jenny said, "She does that with me too. She does it with everyone that showers her. If you'll do Betty, I'll do two of yours. I can't handle her today."

"Okay," I told her.

Then came about the most interesting shower I had given anybody in the twenty years I worked in aged care.

Betty screamed, punched, slapped, and scratched. And also, although I'm not quite sure how I managed it, got showered. At the same

Memories from the Dementia Ward

time, I think more water might have gone on me than on her.

There was a lot of, "Help, help! Murder! Rape!" the entire time I showered her.

Then with the shower finished I got her dry, moisturised, and dressed. By that time, I was sweating and felt like I had just done a circuit class.

Almost done.

I brushed her hair and just as I finished, she grabbed my right arm by the wrist and elbow, lifted my arm to her mouth, and bit me as hard as she possibly could. Then she threw my arm down and said, "There, take that."

I held out my hand with her top and bottom dentures and asked, "Would you like to put your teeth in now?"

She took her teeth and put them in then patted my arm saying, "Thank you, dear. That was wonderful."

As I walked her out of her room to take her to breakfast, a group of people stood open-mouthed in the hallway—the facility owner with a group of prospective customers.

By the look of them, it was clear they had heard the screaming.

A couple of times in the following week, I listened in when the girls were showering Betty, and she did just as

Memories from the Dementia Ward

much screaming. And there was also just as much punching, slapping, and scratching as there had been with me.

I still felt uncomfortable showering her.

Edward Spellman

Memories from the Dementia Ward

Punched in the Face
Mr David Morgan

David was a small man and a boxer in his time.

"A champion flyweight," he told me. There were newspaper clippings of him in his boxing shorts and gloves on his wall.

One day, I was getting David ready for bed using the hoist which required two staff. While I waited for my partner, I put his pyjama top on. I stood directly in front of him at the time and never did that again with David.

As I was doing up his buttons, he snapped into fight mode. The fists came up and he gave me a good one right on the chin before I could react.

The first punch was followed by two or three more, which all missed because I had leant back after the first one and he was sitting in his princess chair.

He had his guard up as he ducked and weaved from side to side saying, "I can take you."

He grinned from ear to ear.

Memories from the Dementia Ward

I held my hands up, palms open. I said, "You win David."

That made him laugh and there was a sparkle in his eyes that hadn't been there before.

After that episode, he became more animated and friendly, at least to me. I would put my fists up to him and say, "Come on, Dave, I'll have ya."

He loved it and seemed to think my putting my fists up to him was hilarious. I'm pretty sure I was holding them all wrong.

He would throw a few shadow punches and laugh but he never hit me again. He never even tried, although

Edward Spellman

other staff members had a bit of a hard time with him and were hit.

Memories from the Dementia Ward

Strawberry Jam
Mrs Joan Sanderson

Dinner time in the dementia ward got hectic at times. And at those times, it was not uncommon to miss something. Which I did.

The evening meal had finished, and we were taking people back to their rooms to get them ready for bed. I started by taking the residents in princess chairs back to their rooms first to wait until there were two of us to put them to bed.

On this particular night, I had just come back into the dining room after taking the last resident in a princess chair back to her room.

The next resident to take back was Joan who was a diabetic. At her table, there were three other residents. Joan and one other were in wheelchairs, while the other were ambulant on their own.

The residents got attached to their places in the dining room and this group had been sitting together for about six months. The woman beside Joan had

Memories from the Dementia Ward

her jar of strawberry jam that was kept in the kitchen fridge and only brought out for her at mealtimes. When I returned to the dining room, the jar was on the table in front of Joan. Empty. With a dessert spoon sticking out of it. It was a rather large jar.

When I had opened it for Mrs Sanderson at the beginning of the meal, it had been full.

Not anymore. Joan had eaten the whole jar of strawberry jam and there was more jam on Joan's face than was left in the jar.

"Why did you eat the jam?" I asked her.

"Wasn't me."

It was my fault for not removing it before I left the dining room.

Then I noticed something in her lap. Twelve empty sweetener sachets. She had eaten the contents.

That was a first and luckily it wouldn't do her any harm.

Ten minutes later when we were changing Joan for bed, we found another ten sachets, intact, stuffed in her bra.

Memories from the Dementia Ward

Folding in the Dark
Mrs Gwen Stapleton

Mrs Stapleton was in a room close to the nurse's station and needed regular checks in case she fell out of bed, which she had done several times.

A small woman of ninety years, she only came up to my shoulder and I'm only 165 cm tall.

I had put her to bed half an hour earlier, so I thought I had better check.

When I opened her bedroom door, a little light from the hallway shined in and I could usually see her in the bed, if she was in the bed.

This time, when I opened the door a little bit and very quietly, Gwen wasn't in the bed.

I opened the door a little more and turned on the bedroom light.

She was standing at the foot of the bed wearing a cheeky grin.

The cheeky grin was the only thing Gwen was wearing. She had stripped both herself and the bed.

Stacked impeccably on the end of the bed, folded perfectly, was all of her bedding. Bedspread, blankets, top sheet, bottom sheet, plastic mac, draw sheet, and pillowcase. Her nightgown, net pants, and pad folded neatly on top of the pile.

I redressed her and sat her in her chair while I remade the bed.

Her folding was impressive because her room was very dark when she did it.

Then I put her back to bed, turned out the lights, closed the door and went off to finish my paperwork.

About twenty minutes later I went to check on her again.

Edward Spellman

I followed the same procedure as I had earlier, opening the door just a little.

Mrs Stapleton was not in her bed…again.

I turned on the light, again, and there was Gwen in almost the same place she had been earlier. Wearing the same cheeky grin, and nothing else.

The bed had been stripped. Gwen had stripped. And everything was neatly folded and stacked on the end of her bed. Again.

So, I redressed her and remade the bed. Then I put her back to bed, turned out the lights and closed the door.

Twenty-five minutes later we went through the whole process all over again, and then again just before my shift finished.

I was pretty sure I couldn't fold things that precisely in the dark.

Edward Spellman

Memories from the Dementia Ward

Scooching Along the Corridor Floor
Mr Patrick Kelly

Gentleman Pat. Pat had gone downhill about a year and a half after he moved into the dementia ward.

Pat lived in Room 9 and I could see down the entire length of the corridor from just outside the office door. The corridor had handrails running along both walls and vinyl on the floor—easier to clean. And in this environment, being easier to clean was definitely a good thing.

I was in the office filling out the bowel charts when I heard a noise I didn't recognise. I rolled out the door on the office chair and looked down the corridor for a look. It was Pat.

Most of the lights were off so I couldn't see him very well. I could tell that he was sitting on the floor in the middle of the corridor. Naked it seemed.

The main light switches were right next to the office door, so I turned on the corridor lights, grabbed a pair of

Memories from the Dementia Ward

rubber gloves as I went down to see what he was up to.

I had only gotten halfway to him when I turned back and retrieved a mop and bucket from the pan room. Then I returned to check on Pat who was further down the corridor than he had been before.

I needed the mop and bucket because Pat had left a trail of faeces along the corridor as he scooched along the floor on his bum.

Is there such a word as scooched? I wasn't sure but it worked for that occasion.

Edward Spellman

Pat was naked and moving himself along the floor. Pulling with his legs and lifting and pushing with his arms while pooing, leaving smeared trail of faeces all the way to his bedroom.

The first thing I did was mop up the poo because it would have been almost impossible to get Pat back into his room without at least one of us stepping in it.

Having mopped up, at least most of it, I then got a couple of face washers, wet them, and went back to Pat.

Memories from the Dementia Ward

"Can I see your hands, Pat?" I asked him.

Pat ignored me and kept scooching down the corridor, leaving his trail.

I cleaned his hands to make sure the was no poo on them. Then turned him around to face the wall and said, "Can you grab the handrail, Pat?"

I guided his hands to the handrail and he grabbed hold.

"Can you pull yourself up, Pat?"

Pat pulled himself up. Which made my life so much easier.

As soon as he stood up, I gave his bum a bit of a wash. Surprisingly it was not very dirty.

Then I walked him back to his room and sat him on the toilet. I changed my gloves and then put on his singlet and pyjama top. I grabbed a plastic bag to put the dirty face washers in and went and picked them up from where I had left them in the corridor.

I checked on Pat, who was still sitting on the toilet.

I went back out and finished mopping up the trail of poo.

Then checked on Pat. Still there.

Memories from the Dementia Ward

I dried the corridor floor then got Pat a pair of net pants a clean pad, and his pyjama trousers.

I slipped on the net pants, put the pad in, and then put on the pyjama bottoms. After that, I put his slippers on.

Pat sat quietly, waiting for me.

Next, I checked his bed, which was clean. It just needed a little tidying up.

Then back into Pat again. I said, "Have you finished Pat?"

No response.

"Can you stand up for me please Pat?"

No response again, so I helped to start the process. Pat then realised what I was up to and stood up.

"Hold onto the sink please, Pat," I said as I guided his hands to the edge of the sink.

If I didn't do that with Pat, he would pull his trousers up as soon as he was standing, giving you no time to clean his bum.

Gentleman Pat held onto the sink while I finished cleaning him up. Then I pulled up his net pants, adjusted his pad, and pulled up his pyjama bottoms.

Memories from the Dementia Ward

I looked in the toilet. Bowels opened. A large four for Pat. And flushed it away.

I walked Pat back to his bed, helped him in, pulled up his blankets, turned off the light, and went back to the office to update Pat's bowel report.

Edward Spellman

Memories from the Dementia Ward

Cornering a Visitor in the Foyer
Miss Elizabeth Acker (Lizzy)

As I walked past the foyer on my way to the pan room, one of the resident's daughters waved to me. She seemed to be talking to another one of the residents, Lizzy.

I waved back and went into the pan room, dropped off the dirty clothes I was carrying and headed past the foyer again on my way down the hallway.

Five minutes later I came back past the foyer and this time Mrs Allan's daughter Mary called out, "Help!"

Whoops. I spun around to see what was wrong.

Lizzy had her back to me and was facing Mary who mouthed, "Help. She won't let me out of the building."

Lizzy seemed to have taken a liking to Mary and wouldn't let her past. She was right up in her face. Barely a hands breadth away and saying, "Glok glok glok glok glok glok glok," and moving to block her every time she tried to get past. The Glok glok glok was constant. I had been in that

Memories from the Dementia Ward

same position with Lizzy from time to time.

Mary was starting to freak out by the look of her so I distracted Lizzy by asking about her boys. She enjoyed talking about them and it gave Mary a chance to slip away.

As she left, she mouthed, "Thank you."

Edward Spellman

Memories from the Dementia Ward

Fake Fainting in the Hallway
Miss Elsa Green

Elsa liked to faint. Or perhaps I should say, that Elsa liked to pretend to faint and had a pretty decent repertoire of faints at her disposal. One for every occasion.

Elsa had spent her working life as a schoolteacher. She sorted me out with her walking stick on several occasions for not doing as I was told—like when

I wouldn't go back to my classroom, often with the threat of detention.

Elsa could walk quite well on her own although she did always use a walking stick. Whenever she saw a staff member or visitor moving in her direction, she would start to swoon. She would sway on her feet, saying, "Oh, oh, help. I'm going to faint."

Then she flailed about with the hand not connected to her walking stick, while closing her eyes, and grabbed hold of anyone within reach.

If I let her grab hold of me, she would flop all of her weight onto me

Memories from the Dementia Ward

and she was not a particularly small woman.

Sometimes she allowed me to help her to the nearest seat. At other times, she grabbed hold of the handrail and go ever so slowly to the floor, decrying, "I'm fainting. I'm fainting."

If Elsa allowed me to help her to the nearest chair where she could rest, she would only sit as long as I stayed with her. Doing the swooning thing sitting down. Then, as soon as I left, she would get up and walk away.

More than once, I had visitors come to me in a panic asking for me to call an ambulance for the poor woman who had just collapsed. I would go with them to see this poor collapsed woman who had often mysteriously recovered as soon as her audience had left. Swooning and fainting was simply how Elsa worked her way through the day.

I had more than one complaint made against me for not calling an ambulance for her when all she needed, or wanted, was a little attention, and perhaps a cup of tea.

My favourite faint of all time was pretty cool I thought. I was heading into a room to make a bed when Elsa was in the corridor just outside that room, and entered full swoon mode.

Memories from the Dementia Ward

One hand went to the handrail, and the back of the other went to her forehead.

"Help, help, I'm going to faint!" she said, her eyes squeezed shut. Flailing with her other hand, she reached for the handrail. Once she had a good solid hold of it, she carefully and slowly lowered herself to the floor while calling out, "I'm fainting. I'm fainting."

"That's nice, Elsa," I said and went into the room and made the bed where I could see her the whole time.

As I left the room, I stepped around her and asked, "Would you like a cup of tea?"

"Oh, that would be nice." She got up off the floor as though she were about forty years younger than her ninety-seven years and came with me to have her cup of tea.

She didn't need any help at all to get up off the floor—pretty good for her age.

Memories from the Dementia Ward

Hiding in the Wardrobe
Mrs Nora Brown and Mrs Gwen Stapleton

During another nightly routine, I was getting another resident ready for bed, Nora. She was sitting on her toilet for a few minutes while I was getting the bed ready and turning down the covers. I checked there was a draw sheet and plastic mac then picked out a night dress fresh pad from the wardrobe.

While I was doing that I heard, or thought I heard, a metallic rattle. It was only for a split second. And then the sound was gone. I listened carefully. Nothing. Perhaps I had imagined it.

While getting Nora changed for bed, I heard it again. This time, I thought it had come from the wardrobe, which was silly. I realised that it was probably the resident in the next room fiddling about in his wardrobe which backed onto this one.

I heard the noise another couple of times and decided to check on the next-door neighbour once Nora was settled. He was notorious for taking all

Memories from the Dementia Ward

of his clothes out of the wardrobe and drawers and piling them on his bed, telling us that he was packing for a trip to the hospital. He often waited for an ambulance and I spent a lot of time putting his clothes back where they belonged.

As I walked Nora out of the bathroom and toward her bed, we passed her wardrobe. One of the doors slid open and Gwen Stapleton peeked out from between a bunch of wire coat hangers with her cheeky grin in place.

Fully clothed this time.

Edward Spellman

Memories from the Dementia Ward

No Sleep

Mr Theo Ruiz (Sophia's son)

Some of the residents in the dementia ward had phones in their rooms while others did not. The phones were organised by the families of the residents and it could be very beneficial for both the resident and their loved ones and it could also cause some trouble.

On a Wednesday afternoon just after entering the ward, I heard shouting coming from Room 17. I knocked on the door and opened it to see if there was anything I could do to help.

Mrs Ruiz was yelling at her son Theo and when I poked my head in the door, I could see from his expression that he was frustrated and angry.

Theo asked if we could talk. We both left the room and went to one of the small sitting rooms. Theo was a contractor who worked in the building industry.

Theo apologised for yelling, then he said, "Mum's driving me crazy. I don't know what to do."

Memories from the Dementia Ward

His mother, Sophia, had been calling her friends and relatives in the middle of the night, who then called Theo and demanded that he get his mother to stop it. Theo had asked his mum not to call people in the middle of the night and she was yelling at him, saying she would call whoever she wanted, whenever she wanted, and that he was a horrible son.

I could see that hurt him deeply. He loved his mum and visited at least twice a week. He always asked us if she needed anything and would get it straight away if she did.

He told me he was not getting any sleep between his mum calling him all hours of the night and calls from her relatives and friends demanding that he do something about this. They didn't mind the daytime calls.

"Can you do anything?" he asked me.

"The only thing I can think of right now would be to disconnect your mum's phone, or to make it so she can only receive calls."

Theo screwed up his face. "I can't do that to Mum. I'll just have to hope she calms down I guess."

Memories from the Dementia Ward

Three days later, Theo came in looking rather ragged. He visited his mum and when he left, he took the phone with him, saying, "I need a couple of nights to sleep."

"There's another option," I told him. "You could have the phone set up to accept incoming calls only. Then she could still get her phone calls and you guys could get your sleep. You would just have to call the phone company and have them set it up."

"I'll look into it tomorrow."

Theo checked it out and had the phone company set it all up so that his mum could still get incoming phone calls but couldn't call out. That way he could get some sleep.

I didn't see Theo again for about two weeks but when I did, he looked rested and in a good space. He told me that the incoming call-only system was working like magic. There were no more late-night phone calls. No more angry relatives and friends calling him. His mum had adapted after just a few days and was getting enough phone calls to keep her happy.

That might not sound like much, but it was pretty intense for Theo and his mum, as well as their friends and relatives who were in the middle of it.

Memories from the Dementia Ward

Fifty Cents
Mrs Bonnie Allan

This story is about my favourite little Scottish lady named Bonnie. And a cute little Scottish lady named Bonnie should always have a best friend called Bell to have tea with. And biscuits. We can't forget the biscuits. Or else. I had forgotten once or twice and there was hell to pay.

Bonnie would come up to me, take her purse out of her bag, and then ask me how much it would cost to buy a cup of tea for both her and her friend Bell.

"It's free, Bonnie. All part of the service."

"Ach noo," Bonnie would say in her thick Scottish accent. "I kenna take it for free. I'll gi ya fifty cent."

I would accept her money and make her and Bell a cup of tea. Bell would drink hers and Bonnie would leave hers until it was cold and then complain that I had given her a cold cup of tea. So, I would remake Bonnie's tea and Bell would complain that it wasn't

Memories from the Dementia Ward

fair that Bonnie was getting a cup of tea and she wasn't.

As soon as a cup of tea arrived, both of them would complain about the lack of biscuits. Which were on their way because I knew how much trouble I would get into if these two didn't get a biscuit or two with their cup of tea.

I would keep the fifty-cent piece Bonnie used to pay for the tea until she wasn't paying attention and then I would slip it back into her purse. That one coin paid for cups of tea for a couple of years until I switched it for another one.

Edward Spellman

I rather liked Bonnie and the way she would buy tea for her friend and herself so after swapping the coins, I kept hers as a memento.

Memories from the Dementia Ward

A Trail of Poo

Mr Peter Smith

The office was a quiet place to sit and I liked to get to work early so I could relax while drinking a cup of tea. It turned out to be not one of those days, although I did get there half an hour before my shift started.

I entered the code into the keypad, stepped through and into the facility, and noticed the scent of poo in the air. I looked down and saw a trail leading from the small lounge room to my left and down the corridor.

The trail looked uncannily familiar, and I suspected who would be at the other end of it. The small lounge room was one of his favourite spots to sit during the afternoon. Luckily, the trail of poo was fresh and had not dried yet as there's nothing worse than trying to clean up dried poo. However, if we had to, or it was on a person, we used shaving cream. It's surprising at how well it cleans up dried poo.

I checked the little lounge and found poo on the chair where the trail began then went and dropped my lunch

Memories from the Dementia Ward

bag off in the office and put on some rubber gloves.

I started at the beginning, cleaning off the chair and spraying the room around it with air freshener.

Then I went to the cleaner's room where I collected a mop and bucket. I followed the trail, mopping as I went. The trail led from the small lounge into the dining room. It went around one dining room table. Then another, and another, before heading off into the other corridor.

I returned to the cleaner's room, emptied my bucket and refilled it with fresh cleaner. I changed my gloves as well.

I realised that I had forgotten to put out some Wet Floor signs, so I grabbed a couple and put two in the corridor, and another in the dining room.

I went back to mopping and headed out of the dining room and into the corridor, mopping along the way and spraying the air freshener around as I went.

As I turned into the second corridor, I saw Mrs Flowers limping along, so I took her to her room, took

Memories from the Dementia Ward

off her shoes and checked inside. Mrs Flowers did not usually limp.

I found someone's bottom dentures wrapped in a tissue and stuffed into the toe of her shoe. Her own dentures were in her mouth.

The dentures in the shoe were also named and had belonged to Mrs Flowers's neighbour who had passed away several months earlier. I took her back out to the lounge room to watch television and noticed Mrs Ruttledge was wearing a nice pair of glasses that had those floral wings at the side of the frame—Mrs Ruttledge didn't wear glasses.

Edward Spellman

I took the glasses to the office and left them on the table with a note. "Does anyone know who these belong to?" Hopefully one of the other staff members would recognise them. Otherwise, they would just end up in the lost glasses' drawer, a bit like the dimension where the other sock goes, or pens that still have ink.

Having sorted out Mrs Flowers limp, I returned to my mopping.

I found myself at Peter's room, 13, where he was sitting on his bed. He had the linen trolley, which had been full of clean linen for the shift but wasn't any longer as he had used most of it trying to clean himself up, creating more mess than when he had started.

As I had found the source, a harsh metallic smell caught in the back of my throat. Poo had been running down his legs and filled his slippers. The overflow was what had made the trail as he shuffled down the corridor. The trail of poo went from one end of the building to the other.

I cleaned Peter's slippers as best I could, then bagged them and sent them to the laundry.

I took Peter into the bathroom and sat him on the toilet before going out to finish moping the hallway and bedrooms.

The trail of poo had gone past his room and into the next room along and diagonally opposite his. Room 14. Then the trail came out of 14 and into 15. Then out of 15 and into 16. Then from 16 back to 13.

With the mopping finished, I returned to Peter's room and showered him, got him dressed in clean clothes and took him out to the lounge room. I took the mop and bucket along with the air freshener back to the cleaner's room and picked up a linen skip for the dirty clothes and towels.

Memories from the Dementia Ward

When I found him in his room, Peter had already used up almost all of the spare linen that should have lasted the entire shift. I filled four large black plastic bags and restocked the trolley or I wouldn't have the linen I needed later in the shift.

I took Peter out to the lounge/dining room to watch television while I went back to set up the rooms for the night. I went to each room, turned down the bed, ensured plastic macs and draw sheets were in place and replace them if they were not. Sometimes the morning shift did not have what they needed, and the linen was not delivered until about half an hour after my shift started.

I closed the windows, turned on the ceiling fans, and air conditioners if necessary. I made sure everyone had pyjamas or a night dress and the appropriate pad.

When I got to the room across the hall from Peter's where the poo trail had led, I turned back the bedspread and found that he had sat on the bed and gotten poo on the blanket. He must have turned the bedspread back as it was clean.

I stripped the blanket off the bed and found the sheet underneath also had

Memories from the Dementia Ward

poo on it. Then the draw sheet, the plastic mac, and the bottom sheet as well. Another full bag of dirty linen.

I emptied that skip and replaced the bag for the next lot of dirty linen, took it back to the pan room and got back to work.

The same mess had been made in the next room, and the next, and in his room as well. Four complete bed strips and remakes, just in case I had a spare minute or two. Which I didn't.

I missed giving the residents their afternoon tea completely that day. By the time I had time to give it to them, it was time to toilet the residents and get them ready for dinner.

Just breathe.

When it came time to put Peter to bed that day, I found him sitting in the recliner in the back corner of Room 14 wearing a nice summer frock. The name tag told me he had taken it out of the wardrobe from the same room. The colour didn't really suit him.

Memories from the Dementia Ward

Gwen Peeing in my Glove
Mrs Gwen Stapleton

Late one night, I was getting Mrs Stapleton ready for bed. She had been sitting on the toilet and had done a wee so I stood her up and reached down with both hands, my right hand at the front and my left at the back, and took hold of her net pants to pull them up.

I was wearing rubber gloves as we always did when attending to a resident's hygiene, to keep our skin clean.

But—and I'd supposed there had to be a but.

Not that time.

As I reached down to pull up her pants she peed again. Her aim was perfect.

She peed onto the inside of my right wrist and filled up my right-hand glove.

It was very neat and she hardly missed a drop. The only thing that got wet, and warm, was my hand.

Memories from the Dementia Ward

Don't you mean Paul
Mrs Surita Ghumman

Looking around the dining room, I saw that everyone had finished their evening meals and had a drink. The wanderers were growing restless and my shift partner was guiding a few of them to the TV area. Then she would start toileting the ambulant residents while I organised those who were in princess chairs. Sometimes we had everyone in bed by 8:30. At other times,

10:30 came and there were still two or three to go.

Surita was going to be first in bed. If she fell sleep in her princess chair, then woke up, she would not go back to sleep once in bed. Indian and weighing a little under forty kilos, Surita had severe arthritis. Her fingers and legs were stiff and painfully atrophied so she didn't like being moved.

I went over to her and asked, "Are you ready for bed Surita?"

Surita stroked the back of my hand. "What's your name?" Surita asked with her beautiful accent.

"My name's Edward."

Memories from the Dementia Ward

"Don't you mean Paul?" she asked.

"My mother told me it's Edward."

She looked up at me, still stroking the back of my hand. "Yes, Paul."

I pushed her princess chair to her room and closed the door to get her ready for bed. As I came around from behind her she asked again, "What's your name?"

I laughed and said, "Edward."

"Don't you mean Paul?"

I repeated, smiling, "My name's Edward, Surita."

She looked at me like she thought there was definitely something wrong with me.

As I prepared to lift Surita into bed with the hoist, she berated me severely in Hindi, with lots of waving and pointing her crooked finger at me. Halfway between the princess chair and her bed, Surita dangled in the hoist sling. She glared at me and said, "Jesus is going to give you such a kicking."

I think that was the best insult I ever had in my entire life.

I finished putting her to bed, changed her into a fresh nightie and

Memories from the Dementia Ward

changed her pad. All the while being berated in Hindi.

"Good night, Surita."

She beckoned me forward with her finger and said, "Come here, Paul. Let me give you a kiss."

I leaned forward.

She gave me a kiss on the cheek and said, in her beautiful voice, "Thank you, Edward."

Edward Spellman

Memories from the Dementia Ward

Edward Spellman

www.ingramcontent.com/pod-product-compliance
Lightning Source LLC
Chambersburg PA
CBHW061736070526
44585CB00024B/2689